CW00410154

The Essential Keto Diet Cookbook 2019-2020

Lose weight with Quick and Easy Ketogenic Recipes incl. 14 Days Weight Loss Plan

1. Auflage

Rosie Baldridge

Copyright © 2019 by Rosie Baldridge

All rights reserved

All rights for this book here presented belong exclusively to the author.
Usage or reproduction of the text is forbidden and requires a clear consent of the author
in case of expectations.

ISBN-9781692737566

TABLE OF CONTENTS

EXCLUSIVE BONUS!

Get Keto Audiobook for FREE NOW!*

The Ultimate Keto Diet Guide 2019-2020:
How to Loose weight with Quick and Easy Steps

SCAN ME

or go to

www.free-keto.co.uk

*Listen free for 30 Days on Audible (for new members only)

PART 1
KETO EXPLAINED

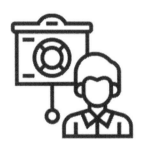

Keto Diet

Recently, the ketogenic diet (keto diet for short), has become quite popular among the general population. Many people see this diet as a way to not only lose weight, but also help them combat a variety of other health issues. The keto diet is a low-carb diet, much like Atkins, in which you get most of your calories from fat and protein instead of carbs. In this type of diet, you cut back significantly on the simple carbs that are easily digested, such as white bread, sugars, sodas, and pastries.

What is "Keto"?

The term "keto" describes a diet that allows your body to produce ketones, which is a molecule that can be used by your body as an alternate energy source when blood sugar/glucose is low. When you consume few simple carbs and a moderate amount of protein, your body produces these molecules.

Ketones are produced by your liver from fat and then used as a fuel source, especially in your brain. Your brain is always busy, consuming vast amounts of energy and can't run on fat- it needs glucose or ketones.

When you decide to try a keto diet, you must be aware that your body will be reliant on fat. This means that your body is in fat-burning mode all day every day. This fat-burning will increase when your insulin levels are low because it's easier to access/burn off the fat stores. While this is a wonderful thing when you're trying to lose weight- there are a few other benefits as well, such as a constant supply of energy and less hunger, which means you stay more focused and alert.

When your body is producing these ketones, you are in a metabolic state that is known as ketosis. The quickest way to get to ketosis is to fast- but it's not the best idea because no one can fast forever. Another way to promote ketosis in your body is the keto diet. This is something that can be done indefinitely. It has the benefits of fasting (weight loss) without having to deprive yourself of food.

KETOSIS: WHAT IS IT?

When you are on a keto diet, your body goes into ketosis. This is basically your body's "survival mode" when food intake has been decreased. Your liver begins to break down the fats stored in it, forming ketones. The primary goal of the keto diet is to force yourself into this state by starving your body of carbs- not calories.

Our bodies are perplexing, they are able to adapt to what we provide them. If we decrease our carb consumption and overload them with fats, it begins to burn ketones for energy. This will give you many amazing benefits, including overall mental and physical health benefits, such as weight loss and increased performance.

How to Lose Weight Effectively on the Keto Diet

We all know that eating in moderation, eating low fat, and decreasing our caloric intake are all effective ways to lose weight. However, these just don't seem to be working very well for most people. If you are one of those who are still trying to lose weight and keep it off, it's time to consider the keto diet.

According to most dietary and health experts, the keto diet is a great way to shed those unwanted pounds. There are lots of people out there who have found this to be true. In this chapter, we'll look at a few tips that can help you effectively lose weight on this diet, as well as some tips to get you started.

Before we delve too deep into the world of keto, you must be aware that this is not an easy way out. If you are hoping for the "magic formula" to shed that extra weight, this is not it.

You'll find that it's easy to fall into the low-carb junk food trap when you're on keto. You must avoid doing this. You want to avoid eating a lot of low carb breads, sugar-free desserts, and pizza.

Okay, with all that being said, it can be scary to start a new diet/new way of life, so here are five steps that can help you get started on the keto diet in a healthy way.

Start preparing yourself now.

Do something to move yourself in the right direction. Find a keto foods list and download it. In the next chapter, we'll take a look at how you can prepare yourself for the keto diet. Ideally, you should start in a week that is not so stressful because it is going to take a bit of prep, both around your home and mentally. If now is not the best time, go ahead and put it on your calendar, so that you're more likely to follow through.

CLEAR OUT FRIDGE AND PANTRY.

When you start any new diet plan/lifestyle change, such as keto, one of the very first things you must do to facilitate your success is to clear out all possible temptation from your fridge and pantry. You're going to have those days where you have zero motivation to continue on your journey. However, if those temptations are not there, it's easier to stick to it.

RESTOCK FRIDGE AND PANTRY WITH KETO-FRIENDLY FOODS.

If keto is something that you're committed to, you must make sure that you have healthy keto options available. So, after you get rid of all the non-keto foods from your fridge and pantry, it's time to restock. Below, you will find a few options:

- All meats
- Seafood/fish
- Eggs
- Nuts/seeds
- Healthy fats (ghee, lard, olive oil, tallow, coconut oil, and avocado oil)
- Leafy greens
- Fruits such as berries and avocado

BE READY FOR THE "KETO FLU"

If you have been consuming a diet high in sugars and carbs, you're probably going to experience what is known as the "keto flu." This is basically because your body is detoxing from all that unhealthy junk and starting to burn fat instead of sugar. Some symptoms of "keto flu" include the following: headaches, fatigue, dizziness, and hunger. This is how you can know that your body is clearing out all those carbs. Another common reason you might experience these symptoms is because you're lacking in electrolytes.

Here are some tips for overcoming "keto flu":

1. Increase fat intake- but not too much. If you have not been eating high amounts of fats, it could be that your digestive system is having difficulty adjusting.
2. Increase calories by adding more eggs, leafy greens, and fatty fish or meats.
3. Include some clean carbs such as root veggies in your diet to facilitate your transition into the keto lifestyle.
4. Get plenty salt by adding salt to your foods and eating foods that are high in potassium, such as leafy greens and avocados.
5. Increase water intake, as dehydration can sometimes be the cause of fatigue, headaches, and nausea.
6. Get some exercise, if possible, which will help your body to become more metabolically flexible and transition to a fat burner quickly. Of course, you must consult with your physician to make sure it's safe for you to exercise.

Find some support.

As you have seen, switching to a keto lifestyle can be quite difficult-even more so when you're doing it all alone. However, if you can get your family and friends to join this lifestyle with you, it will be easier because you can support each other.

However, if your friends and family don't want to join you on your journey, you can find some support on social media. There are plenty of groups on Facebook that can help you on your journey. In addition, there are plenty of keto forums on other social media platforms. You can get the help and information you need- and you can provide/share what you have found to be true for you.

PART 2
RECIPES

Breakfast

In this section, you will find 15 low-carb, keto-friendly breakfast recipes.

Keto-Friendly Cereal

Servings: 3 cups | Total Time: 35 minutes
Nutrition Information
Calories: 801 | Carbs: 20.5 grams | Fats: 75.2 grams

Ingredients:

- Cooking spray
- 1 cup/128 grams each chopped almonds & walnuts
- ¼ cup/32 grams sesame seeds
- 1 cup/128 grams coconut flakes, unsweetened
- 2 Tablespoons/28 grams each chia & flax seeds
- ½ teaspoon/2.5 grams ground clove
- ¼ cup coconut oil, melted
- 1 teaspoon/5 ml vanilla extract
- 1 ½ teaspoon/7.5 grams cinnamon
- 1 large egg white
- ½ teaspoon/2.5 grams salt

Instructions:

1 Preheat oven to 350°F/176°C.
2 Using cooking spray, grease baking sheet.
3 In a large bowl, combine seeds, coconut flakes, and nuts.
4 Add salt, cloves, vanilla, and cinnamon.
5 Beat egg whites until foamy in a separate bowl. Add the seeds, coconut flakes, and nuts.
6 Add coconut oil and stir until well coated.
7 Spread evenly onto baking sheet and bake for 10 to 12 mins. Stir and place back in oven until golden, about 12 mins.
8 Allow to cool before serving.

Breakfast Sausage Sandwich

Servings: 3 | Total Time: 15 mins
Nutrition Information
Calories: 444 | Carbs: 7.2 grams | Fats: 38.7 grams

Ingredients:

- ◆ 6 eggs
- ◆ Salt & pepper (to taste)
- ◆ Pinch red pepper flakes
- ◆ 2 Tablespoons heavy cream
- ◆ 3 slices cheese (your choice)
- ◆ Sliced avocado
- ◆ 1 Tablespoon butter
- ◆ 6 frozen sausage patties (follow package directions for prep)

Instructions:

1 Beat together eggs, cream, and red pepper flakes in a small bowl. Season as you wish with salt/pepper.

2 Place skillet over medium heat to melt butter.

3 Pour 1/3 of eggs in skillet and place a slice of cheese in the middle.

4 Cook for approximately one minute.

5 Fold egg in half, covering the cheese. Remove from pan and repeat with the rest of the eggs.

6 Take 2 sausage patties and place avocado and egg in between, making a sandwich.

Cabbage Hashbrowns

Servings: 2 | Total Time: 25 mins
Nutrition Information
Calories: 157 | Carbs: 6.3 grams | Fats: 11.9 grams

Ingredients:

- 2 large eggs
- ½ teaspoon each garlic powder & salt
- 2 cup cabbage, shredded
- Black pepper (to taste)
- 1 Tablespoon vegetable oil
- ¼ small yellow onion, thin sliced

Instructions:

1 Whisk together eggs, garlic powder, and salt. Sprinkle black pepper if you wish.

2 Add cabbage and onions and toss together.

3 On medium high heat, heat oil in large skillet.

4 Divide cabbage mixture into 4 patties and place in hot oil.

5 Use spatula to flatten.

6 Cook until tender and golden, about 3 mins on each side.

Breakfast Cups

Servings: 12 | Total Time: 40 mins
Nutrition Information
Calories: 250 | Carbs: 1.2 grams | Fats: 13.3 grams

Ingredients:

- 2 pounds pork, ground
- ½ teaspoon each cumin and paprika
- Salt/Pepper (to taste)
- 1 Tablespoon each fresh chopped thyme and chives
- 2 cup shredded cheese (your choice)
- 2 garlic cloves, minced
- 2 ½ cup chopped fresh spinach
- 1 dozen eggs

Instructions:

1 Preheat oven to 400°F/204°C
2 Combine pork with garlic, cumin, salt, thyme, paprika, and black pepper.
3 Place a small amount of pork mixture into each muffin tin well and press up sides to make a cup.
4 Evenly divide cheese and spinach between pork cups.
5 Crack an egg on top and season with salt/pepper to taste.
6 Bake for about 25 mins, until eggs are set and sausage is cooked through.

Blueberry Muffins

Servings: 12 (1 dozen muffins) | Total Time: 40 mins
Nutrition Information
Calories: 70 | Carbs: 1.7 grams | Fats: 6.25 grams

Ingredients:

- ½ teaspoon each salt and baking soda
- 1 ½ teaspoon baking powder
- 1/3 cup keto-friendly sweetener
- 1 teaspoon vanilla extract
- 2 ½ cups almond flour
- 3 large eggs
- 1/3 cup each melted butter and unsweetened almond milk
- 2/3 cup blueberries
- Optional: zest from ½ lemon

Instructions:

1 Line 12-cup muffing pan with liners, if desired.

2 Preheat oven to 350°F/176°C.

3 In a large bowl, combine almond flour, baking powder, salt, baking soda, and sweetener.

4 Add almond milk, vanilla, eggs, and melted butter until just combined.

5 Fold in blueberries and lemon zest (if desired) until evenly blended.

6 Divide batter evenly among the 12 cups and bake until golden and toothpick comes out clean- about 23 mins.

7 Allow time to cool before serving.

Pepper Omelet Cups

Servings: 4 | Total Time: 1 hour
Nutrition Information
Calories: 370 | Carbs: 6.7 grams | Fats: 26.5 grams

Ingredients:

- 8 eggs
- 2 bell peppers, halved & seeded
- 1 cup cheese, shredded
- ¼ cup milk
- 2 Tablespoons chives, finely chopped
- 4 slices bacon, cooked/ crumbled
- Salt & pepper (to taste)

Instructions:

1 Preheat oven to 400°F/204°C.

2 Put a small amount of water in baking dish and place peppers cut side up. Bake for 5 mins.

3 While peppers are baking, beat together milk and eggs. Add chives, bacon, and cheese. Season with salt and pepper as you wish.

4 When peppers come out of oven, distribute egg mixture evenly.

5 Bake until eggs are set, 35 to 40 mins.

Jalapeno Egg Cups

Servings: 4-6 | Total Time: 35 m**ins**
Nutrition Information
Calories: 394 | Carbs: 2.4 grams | Fats: 29.8 grams

Ingredients:

- 12 slices bacon
- 10 large eggs
- ¼ cup sour cream
- 2 large jalapenos
- ½ cup each cheddar and mozzarella cheeses
- Salt/pepper, to taste
- 1 teaspoon garlic powder

Instructions:

1 Preheat oven to 375°F/190°C.
2 In large skillet, slightly cook bacon- until brown but pliable. Set aside to drain.
3 Whisk together eggs, cheeses, garlic powder, sour cream, and minced jalapeno.
4 Season as desired with salt/pepper.
5 Spray pan with non-stick cooking spray and line with bacon.
6 Pour egg mixture into each cup and top with jalapeno slice.
7 Bake until eggs appear cooked through, about 20 mins.
8 Allow to cool before serving.

Zucchini Egg Cups

Servings: 12 | Total Time: 40 mins
Nutrition Information
Calories: 119 | Carbs: 2.3 grams | Fats: 8.8 grams

Ingredients:

- 8 eggs
- 2 medium zucchini, peeled into strips
- ½ cup cherry tomatoes, cut into quarters
- ¼ pound ham
- Salt & pepper (to taste)
- ½ cup heavy cream
- ½ teaspoon oregano
- 1 cup cheddar cheese
- 1 pinch red pepper flakes

Instructions:

1 Preheat oven to 400°F/204°C.
2 Spray muffin tin with cooking spray.
3 Line muffin tin wells with zucchini strips to create a crust.
4 Sprinkle cherry tomatoes and ham inside each one.
5 In a separate bowl, whisk together eggs, cream, oregano, and red pepper flakes. Season with salt and pepper as desired.
6 Pour mixture into muffin tin wells and add cheese to top, as desired.
7 Bake until eggs are set, about 30 mins.

Keto Bread

Servings: 1 loaf (multiple servings) | Total Time: 1 hour 10 mins
Nutrition Information
Calories: 101 | Carbs: 1.6 grams | Fats: 9 grams

Ingredients:

- 6 large eggs
- ¼ cup butter, melted & cooled
- ½ teaspoon each cream of tartar and salt
- 1 ½ cup almond flour
- 1 Tablespoon baking powder

Instructions:

1 Line 8x4 loaf pan with parchment paper.

2 Preheat oven to 375°F/190°C.

3 Separate whites and yolks.

4 Combine cream of tartar with egg whites in one bowl and whip until stiff peaks form.

5 In separate bowl, beat together melted butter, egg yolks, salt, baking powder, and almond flour.

6 Fold in whipped egg whites 1/3 at a time until fully incorporated.

7 Pour mixture into pan, making sure the top is smooth.

8 Bake for 30 mins or until slightly golden and toothpick comes out clean.

9 Allow 30 mins of cooling time before slicing/serving.

Avocado Bacon Bombs

Servings: 4 | Total Time: 20 mins
Nutrition Information
Calories: 449 | Carbs: 9.3 grams | Fats: 38.6 grams

Ingredients:

- 2 avocados
- 8 slices bacon
- 1/3 cup cheddar cheese, shredded

Instructions:

1. Turn broiler on oven and line baking sheet with foil.
2. Slice avocados in half, remove pits, and peel skin off.
3. Fill two halves of avocado with cheese (where the pits were), and top with the other half of each.
4. Wrap each one with 4 slices bacon.
5. Place on baking sheet and broil until bacon is slightly crispy, about 5 mins.
6. Using tongs, carefully flip avocado and cook until crispy all over.
7. Cut in half and serve immediately.

Cheesy Ham & Egg Cups

Servings: 12 | Total Time: 25 mins
Nutrition Information
Calories: 148 | Carbs: 1.8 grams | Fats: 9.9 grams

Ingredients:

- Cooking spray
- 1 dozen eggs
- 1 cup shredded cheese
- 12 slices ham
- Salt & pepper (to taste)
- Fresh parsley, chopped (for garnish)

Instructions:

1 Preheat oven to 400°F/204°C.

2 Spray muffin tin with cooking spray and line each cup with ham.

3 Sprinkle with cheddar.

4 Crack 1 egg into each muffin well and season with salt/pepper, as you wish.

5 Bake until eggs are cooked to your personal preference.

6 If you wish, garnish with parsley.

Breakfast Stacks

Servings: 3 | Total Time: 20 mins
Nutrition Information
Calories: 469 | Carbs: 6.2 grams | Fats: 43.1 grams

Ingredients:

- 1 avocado, mashed
- Salt & pepper (to taste)
- 3 breakfast sausage patties
- 3 large eggs
- Hot sauce & chives for garnish, if desired

Instructions:

1. Follow package directions to prepare breakfast sausage.
2. Mash avocado onto sausage and season, as desired, with salt/pepper.
3. Spray cooking spray onto medium skillet and place on medium heat.
4. Spray mason jar lid and place in center of skillet. Crack egg inside lid and season with salt/pepper as desired.
5. Cook until whites are set and remove lid to continue cooking.
6. Place egg on top of sausage/avocado stack.
7. Garnish with hot sauce and chives, if desired.

BEC Roll-Ups

Servings: 6 | Total Time: 20 mins

Nutrition Information

Calories: 552 | Carbs: 2.1 grams | Fats: 43.3 grams

Ingredients:

- 6 large eggs
- Salt & pepper (to taste)
- ¼ teaspoon garlic powder
- 18 slices bacon
- 2 Tablespoons milk
- 2 cups cheese, shredded
- 1 Tablespoon each butter and chopped fresh chives

Instructions:

1 Whisk together eggs, garlic powder, and milk. Season with salt/pepper as desired.

2 In nonstick skillet over medium heat, melt butter.

3 Add eggs and scramble for 3 minutes. Add chives.

4 On cutting board, lay out 3 strips of bacon.

5 Sprinkle cheese on the bottom third and top with some of the eggs.

6 Roll up tightly.

7 Repeat process with remaining Ingredients:.

8 Place skillet back on stove and add the bacon rollups, seam side down.

9 Cook until crisp.

10 Remove from pan to paper towel-lined plate to drain fat.

Breakfast Hash

Servings: 4-6 | Total Time: 50 mins
Nutrition Information
Calories: 217 | Carbs: 9.7 grams | Fats: 14 grams

Ingredients:

- 4 eggs
- 3 Tablespoons water
- 1 cup shredded cheese
- 1 each onion and bell pepper, chopped finely
- 1 cauliflower head, chopped
- Salt & pepper (to taste)
- 2 teaspoons minced garlic
- 2 Tablespoons chives
- ¼ teaspoon paprika

Instructions:

1   Fry bacon until crispy in a large skillet on medium heat. Remove bacon and place on a paper towel lined plate to drain. Leave bacon grease in pan.

2   Add bell pepper, onion, and cauliflower to bacon grease and cook until veggies begin to turn golden and soften. Season with salt, pepper, and paprika.

3   Add water and cover. Cook until water has evaporated and cauliflower is tender. If the water evaporates before the cauliflower is tender, add more water and re-cover.

4   Remove lid and stir in garlic and chives. Cook for about 30 seconds.

5   Use a wooden spoon to make holes in the cauliflower. Crack one egg into each void. Season with salt/pepper, as desired.

6   Sprinkle with bacon and cheese.

7   Put lid on skillet and cook until eggs are to your liking.

Breakfast Bake with Cauliflower

Servings: 6 | Total Time: 55 mins
Nutrition Information
Calories: 430 | Carbs: 6.8 grams | Fats: 31.2 grams

Ingredients:

- 10 eggs
- 8 slices bacon
- 1 head of cauliflower
- Salt & pepper (to taste)
- 2 cups cheese, shredded
- 1 cup milk
- 2 green onions, sliced thin
- 1 cup milk
- Optional: hot sauce and green onions for garnish

Instructions:

1 Preheat oven to 350°F/176°C.
2 Place cauliflower into food process and roughly process. Place in baking dish.
3 Top with green onions, cheese, and bacon.
4 In skillet on medium heat, fry bacon until crisp and place on a paper towel-lined plate to drain the excess fat.
5 Whisk together milk, eggs, paprika, garlic, salt, and pepper.
6 Pour egg mixture on top of cauliflower mixture in baking dish.
7 Bake about 35-40 mins, until eggs are set and golden on top.

LUNCH

In this section, you will find 15 low-carb, keto-friendly lunch recipes.

Coleslaw Keto Wraps

Servings: 4 | Total Time: 30 mins
Nutrition Information
Calories: 190 | Carbs: 14.6 grams | Fats: 14.8 grams

Ingredients:

- **Slaw**
- 3 cups red cabbage, thin sliced
- ½ cup green onions, diced
- ¾ cup mayo
- ¼ teaspoon salt
- 2 teaspoons apple cider vinegar
- **Wraps & Additional Filling**
- 16 collard green leaves
- 1 pound ground meat of your choice, cooked/chilled
- 1/3 cup alfalfa sprouts

Instructions:

1 Combine slaw Ingredients:, mixing with a spoon until well coated.

2 Remove stems from collard green leaves and place one on clean surface.

3 Place a spoonful on the far edge. Add a spoonful of meat. Top with sprouts.

4 Roll filling in leaf, making sure to tuck in the sides so the filling does not fall out.

5 After rolling wrap, insert 1-2 toothpicks to hold it together. *This is especially helpful if you're taking your lunch out with you.*

6 Repeat with remaining leaves and filling.

Dijon Herb Salmon Salad

Servings: 4 | Total Time: 35 mins
Nutrition Information
Calories: 484 | Carbs: 10.7 grams | Fats: 29.7 grams

Ingredients:

- **Salmon/Salad**
- 2 eight ounce salmon filets
- Salt & pepper to taste
- ½ cucumber, cut lengthwise and sliced
- 1 tomato, diced
- 2 green onions, chopped thin
- 4 celery sticks, diced
- **Dressing**
- 2 Tablespoons each Dijon mustard, water, olive oil, and lemon juice
- 1 garlic clove
- ¾ teaspoon each rosemary and thyme leaves
- Salt & pepper (to taste)
- 1 teaspoon black mustard seeds
- ¼ cup flat leaf parsley, chopped roughly

Instructions:

1. Turn broiler on and line baking sheet with foil.
2. Place salmon on prepared baking sheet and sprinkle with salt/pepper.
3. Place in oven to broil- about 4 to 5 inches from heat. Should be broiled for about 10 mins per inch of thickness.
4. When salmon is golden brown, remove from oven and set aside to cool.
5. When cool, break apart into large bowl and add celery, tomato, green onions, and cucumber and set aside.
6. Place all dressing Ingredients: into blender and blend until smooth. Pour over salmon/veggie mixture.
7. Serve over greens, straight up, or as a sandwich.

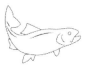

Bacon Wrapped Chicken Tenders

Servings: 8 | Total Time: 45 mins
Nutrition Information
Calories: 768 | Carbs: 2 grams | Fats: 37.7 grams

Ingredients:

- 2 teaspoons each: salt, cayenne pepper (less if you prefer less spice), garlic powder, and paprika
- 1 teaspoon each thyme, onion powder, and oregano
- 16 chicken tenders (about 16)
- 16 slices bacon, no sugar added

Instructions:

1 Preheat oven to 425°F/218°C.
2 Line 2 baking pans with foil and top with metal rack.
3 Place all herbs/spices in a zipper bag and close. Shake to blend.
4 Place each chicken tender in bag and shake to coat.
5 Once coated, wrap in bacon, tucking the ends in. Place on rack in prepared pan.
6 Bake for about 35 mins, or until bacon is crispy.

Bacon and Mushroom Skillet

Servings: 1-2 | Total Time: 20 mins
Nutrition Information
Calories: 231 | Carbs: 5.1 grams | Fats: 16.2 grams

Ingredients:

- 4 slices bacon
- 2 cups mushrooms, halved
- ½ teaspoon salt
- 1 Tablespoon each thyme and garlic confit

Instructions:

1 Place cast iron skillet on stovetop on medium heat.

2 While skillet is heating, prepare Ingredients:.

3 Cut bacon into pieces, about ½" each. Slice mushrooms in ½. If using fresh thyme, remove leaves from stems.

4 Cook bacon until crispy.

5 Move bacon aside and add mushrooms. Sauté until browned and starting to soften.

6 Add thyme, garlic, and salt. Cook for 5 mins, stirring regularly.

7 Once mushrooms have become golden and juicy, remove from heat.

8 Serve on greens or in warm broth.

Keto Cobb Salad

Servings: 2 | Total Time: 35 mins
Nutrition Information
Calories: 665 | Carbs: 24.7 grams | Fats: 32.2 grams

Ingredients:

- 2 ½ cups each, spinach & romaine, chopped
- 2 boneless/skinless chicken breasts
- 2 hard-boiled eggs
- 8 cherry tomatoes, sliced
- 4 slices bacon, cooked
- ¼ onion, chopped fine
- ¼ cup bleu cheese
- 1 Tablespoon lime juice
- Salt/pepper, as desired

Instructions:

1 Preheat oven to 350°F/176°C.

2 Spray baking sheet with non-stick cooking spray.

3 Place chicken on baking sheet and season with salt/pepper, as desired.

4 Cook chicken until internal temp is 165°F/73°C.

5 Slice and set aside.

6 Build salads in 2 bowls by adding greens, chicken, tomatoes, onion, bacon, bleu cheese, and eggs.

7 Drizzle with lime juice (or your choice of dressing), sprinkle with salt & pepper as desired, and toss to combine.

Tuna Pickle Boats

Servings: 12 pickle boats | Total Time: 15 mins
Nutrition Information
Calories: 39 calories | Carbs: 1.9 grams | Fats: 2.4 grams

Ingredients:

- 1 can/pouch (6-ounce) smoked tuna
- 2 cans/pouches (6-ounce each) albacore tuna
- ¼ teaspoon each garlic powder and pepper
- 1/3 cup mayo, sugar free
- ½ teaspoon onion powder
- 6 whole dill pickles

Instructions:

1 Cut pickles in half. Scoop out seeds and set aside.

2 Combine tuna, mayo, and seasonings in medium bowl and mix well.

3 Scoop about 3 Tablespoons of tuna into each pickle half and serve.

Caesar Egg Salad Wraps

Servings: 4 | Total Time: 20 mins
Nutrition Information
Calories: 137 | Carbs: 3.2 grams | Fats: 10.2 grams

Ingredients:

- 6 hardboiled eggs, peeled/ chopped
- 3 Tablespoons each creamy Caesar dressing and mayo
- ½ cup Parmesan cheese
- Black pepper, as desired
- 4 large leaves romaine lettuce

Instructions:

1 In mixing bowl, combine egg, mayo, dressing, pepper, and ½ of the cheese.

2 Spread romaine leaves on plate.

3 Divide mixture among the romaine leaves and top with remainder of cheese, if desired.

Keto Taco Salad

Servings: 8 | Total Time: 25 mins
Nutrition Information
Calories: 1003 | Carbs: 10.8 grams | Fats: 65.8 grams

Ingredients:

Taco Seasoning

- 2 Tablespoons chili powder
- 2 teaspoons each cumin and garlic powder
- 1 teaspoon salt
- ½ teaspoon each onion powder, cayenne pepper, and oregano
- ¼ teaspoon paprika

Taco Salad

- 16 oz ground beef (80/20)
- 8 ounces cheese, Mexican blend
- 1 head lettuce, chopped
- 2 Tablespoons taco seasoning (check recipe above)
- 1 avocado, cubed
- 8 ounces grape tomatoes, cut in half
- 1/3 cup creama (Mexican Cream)
- 8 ounces chopped red onion
- 2 Tablespoons chopped cilantro

Instructions:

1 Place all taco seasoning Ingredients: in jar, tighten lid, and shake until well combined.

2 Cook ground beef on medium-high heat for about 10 mins, or until browned to your preference.

3 Drain excess grease and stir in 2 Tablespoons taco seasoning. Combine and continue to cook for approximately 5 mins.

4 Place remainder of Ingredients: in bowl and add ground beef. Top with cream and cilantro.

Avocado-Chicken-Cucumber Salad

Servings: 6 | Total Time: 10 mins
Nutrition Information
Calories: 224 | Carbs: 11.6 grams | Fats: 20.4 grams

Ingredients:

- rotisserie chicken, deboned/ shredded (remove skin if desired)
- cucumber, cut in ½ lengthwise and then cut into quarter inch slices
- ¼ onion, thin sliced
- 4 or 5 roma tomatoes, chopped or sliced
- Tablespoons olive oil 2 avocados, peeled/pitted/ diced
- Salt & pepper, to taste
- 2-3 tablespoons lemon (or lime) juice
- ½ cup flat leaf parsley, chopped

Instructions:

1 In a large bowl, combine cucumbers, onion, avocados, chicken, tomatoes, and parsley.

2 Drizzle with olive oil and lemon (or lime) juice and season with salt/ pepper as desired.

3 Toss gently to combine flavors.

Zucchini Grilled Cheese

Servings: 2 sandwiches | Total Time: 40-50 mins
Nutrition Information
Calories: 256 | Carbs: 8.9 grams | Fats: 19.2 grams

Ingredients:

- ◆ Zucchini "Bread" Slices
- ◆ 4 cups zucchini, shredded
- ◆ 1 teaspoon oregano
- ◆ 1 egg
- ◆ ½ cup shredded cheese, mozzarella
- ◆ 4 Tablespoons grated Parmesan cheese
- ◆ Salt/pepper, as desired
- ◆ Grilled Cheese Sandwich
- ◆ 1 Tablespoon room temperature butter
- ◆ ½ cup cheddar cheese (room temp), grated or shredded

Instructions:

1. To make zucchini "bread" slices, preheat oven to 450°F/232°C.
2. Place rack in the middle.
3. Line baking sheet with greased parchment paper or silicone baking mat.
4. Place zucchini in microwave-safe dish and microwave for 5 mins on high.
5. Transfer to dishcloth/tea towel and squeeze out moisture- as much as you can. The zucchini must be dry or the "dough" will be too wet and can't be used as bread.
6. In a bowl, combine zucchini, egg, salt/pepper, oregano, and cheeses. Spread on baking sheet, creating four squares.
7. Bake for about 16 to 21 mins, until slightly brown.
8. Allow to cool before gently removing from parchment paper, taking care to avoid breaking them.
9. Heat skillet on medium heat and spread butter on one side of each piece of "bread". Place buttered side down in skillet, top with cheese and then the other slice of "bread" (with buttered side up this time).
10. Turn heat to medium low and cook until golden, about 2 to 4 mins.
11. Flip over and repeat on other side, cooking for 2-4 mins.

Chicken Enchilada Bowl

Servings: 4 | Total Time: 50 mins
Nutrition Information
Calories: 573 | Carbs: 9.4 grams | Fats: 41.1 grams

Ingredients:

- 2 Tablespoons coconut oil
- 1 pound boneless/skinless chicken thighs
- cup water
- ¾ cup red enchilada sauce
- ¼ cup onion, chopped
- 1 (4-ounce) can green chilies, diced
- 1 avocado, diced
- 1 tomato, chopped
- 1 cup shredded cheese
- ¼ cup pickled jalapenos, chopped
- ½ cup sour cream

Instructions:

1 Place coconut oil in pot and turn on medium heat. Once oil is hot, place chicken in and sear lightly.

2 Add enchilada sauce and water, stirring to combine. Then, add green chilis and onions.

3 Decrease heat and cover.

4 Cook until chicken is tender, but cooked through- approximately 18-27 mins. The internal temp should be 165°F/74°C.

5 Remove from pan and place on cutting board. After shredding/chopping, place chicken back in pot and allow to simmer for 10 mins. The sauce will reduce a bit and the flavor will infuse into the chicken.

6 Put chicken on plates and top with sour cream, jalapeno, avocado, tomato, cheese, and other toppings as desired. Serve over cauliflower rice or alone.

Tuna Salad Stuffed Tomatoes

Servings: 1 | Total Time: 10 mins
Nutrition Information
Calories: 427 | Carbs: 4 grams | Fats: 19.5 grans

Ingredients:

- 1 tomato
- 2 teaspoons balsamic vinegar
- 1 Tablespoon each mozzarella (chopped), fresh basil, and green onion
- 1 can tuna, well drained

Instructions:

1 Cut off tomato top and scoop out insides. Then, set aside.
2 Combine tuna, mozzarella, basil, green onion, and tuna in separate bowl.
3 Fill hollowed out tomato with tuna salad.

Salmon/Avocado Sushi Roll

Servings: 1 | Total Time: 10 mins
Nutrition Information
Calories: 850 | Carbs: 82.8 grams | Fats: 41.5 grams

Ingredients:

- 3 seaweed wrappers
- 6 ounces cooked/canned salmon
- 2 Tablespoons mayo
- 1 sprig green onion, diced into small pieces
- 1 Tablespoon hot sauce
- 1/3 red bell pepper, cut into pieces
- ½ avocado, chopped small
- ½ cucumber, chopped small
- 1 teaspoon sesame seeds
- (Optional) coconut aminos to dip

Instructions:

1 Place seaweed wraps shiny side down on a flat surface Notice the direction of the fibers to determine which way to roll it.

2 Add 1/3 of the salmon to the seaweed wrap and top with avocado, pepper, cucumber, and green onion.

3 Drizzle with mayo and hot sauce.

4 Sprinkle with sesame seeds now- or after it's rolled.

5 Lightly wet the top of the seaweed wrap and pick up the outer edge and start tightly wrapping over Ingredients:.

6 Roll until top edge overlaps and press to stick.

7 Once rolled, place on cutting board, seam down and cut into pieces.

Beef Stuffed Peppers

Servings: 3 | Total Time: 40 mins
Nutrition Information
Calories: 325 | Carbs: 11.9 grams | Fats: 13.7

Ingredients:

- 3 bell peppers
- 2/3 cup ground beef
- 12 mushrooms, chopped finely
- 1 teaspoon olive oil
- 2 slices bacon, chopped finely
- 1 teaspoon paprika
- Salt/pepper, as desired

Instructions:

1 Preheat oven to 350°F/180°C.
2 Cut top off bell peppers and remove seeds. Brush olive oil on the inside and outside of peppers and set aside.
3 Heat olive oil in pan and cook bacon until crispy. Remove bacon, but leave oil/grease in pan.
4 Add onion and mushrooms. Cook until soft. Add beef and sprinkle with paprika.
5 Cook until beef is browned. Season with salt/pepper as desired. Add bacon.
6 Remove from heat.
7 Scoop mixture into bell peppers.
8 Place peppers on prepared baking sheet and bake for approximately 26 mins.

Chicken Skewers with Tzatziki Sauce

Servings: 2 | Total Time: 30 mins
Nutrition Information
Calories: 406 | Carbs: 8.7 grams | Fats: 18.9 grams

Ingredients:

Chicken:
- 2 chicken breasts (cut into chunks)
- 1 Tablespoon each olive oil and white wine vinegar
- 1 teaspoon oregano
- ½ teaspoon paprika

Tzatziki Sauce:
- 5 ounces yogurt
- ¼ cucumber, grated
- 2 cloves garlic, peeled/ crushed
- 1 mint leaves, chopped finely
- Salt, to taste

To serve:
- 2 tomatoes, sliced
- Lettuce leaves
- ¼ cucumber, sliced

Instructions:

1 Preheat oven to 400°F/200°C.

2 If you're using wooden skewers, make sure to place them in water to soak for at least 10 mins.

3 Place chicken in bowl and add paprika, oregano, oil, and vinegar- and combine well. Thread chicken onto skewers and place skewers on baking sheet.

4 Bake chicken until cooked through, approximately 20 mins.

5 While chicken is in oven, blend together tzatziki sauce Ingredients: in separate bowl. Serve sauce with chicken.

6 If desired, serve with sliced cucumber, tomatoes, and lettuce leaves.

DINNER

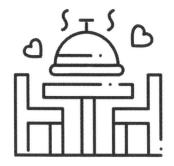

In this section, you will find 15 low-carb, keto-friendly dinner recipes.

Chicken & Broccoli Casserole

Servings: 4 | Total Time: 55 mins
Nutrition Information
Calories: 417 | Carbs: 11.9 grams | Fats: 24.2 grams

Ingredients:

- ◆ 2 Tablespoons coconut oil
- ◆ 4 cups broccoli florets
- ◆ 1 medium white onion (diced)
- ◆ Salt & pepper (to taste)
- ◆ 8 ounces mushrooms
- ◆ 3 cups chicken, cooked and shredded
- ◆ 1 cup each chicken broth and heavy cream or coconut milk
- ◆ 2 eggs
- ◆ (Optional) ½ teaspoon nutmeg

Instructions:

1. Preheat oven to 350°F/180°C.
2. Use 1 Tablespoon of coconut oil to grease casserole dish and set aside.
3. Lightly steam broccoli and set aside, uncovered.
4. Melt coconut oil in saucepan and brown onions. Season with salt/pepper, if you want.
5. Add mushrooms and sauté until cooked through, then move pan off heat.
6. Set pan aside
7. Transfer mushrooms, broccoli, onions, and chicken to the casserole dish.
8. Whisk together salt/pepper, eggs, coconut milk, nutmeg, and broth in separate bowl. Pour mixture into casserole dish.
9. Place in oven and cook 30 to 40 mins, until done in center.

Keto Fried Chicken

Servings: 6 pieces | Total time: 55 mins
Nutrition Information
Calories: 448 | Carbs: 4.1 grams | Fats: 22.2 grams

Ingredients:

- 6 chicken thighs, boneless
- 4 ounces crushed pork rinds
- 2 teaspoons each salt and thyme
- 1 teaspoon garlic powder
- 1 ½ teaspoon paprika
- ¼ teaspoon each cayenne and black peppers
- ¼ cup mayo
- 2 Tablespoons hot sauce
- 1 egg
- 1 Tablespoon mustard

Instructions:

1 Preheat oven to 425°F/218°C

2 Line baking sheet with parchment paper and move rack to top position.

3 Using paper towels, pat chicken dry and set aside.

4 Place dry Ingredients: in bowl and mix well. Transfer half to shallow dish.

5 In separate bowl, combine mayo, mustard, egg, and hot sauce.

6 One at a time, dip chicken thighs in the wet mixture. Then, dip into dry mixture, making sure to flip a few times to ensure chicken is completely covered.

7 Place chicken on baking sheet and bake for 35-41 mins, or until internal temp has reached 165°F/74°C.

Shrimp Stir Fry

Servings: 3-4 | Total Time: 24 mins
Nutrition Information
Calories: 184 | Carbs: 10.1 grams | Fats: 2 grams

Ingredients:

- 1 pound shrimp, peeled/tail on
- 4 green onion stalks
- 2" piece ginger root
- 4 baby portobello mushrooms
- 2 cloves garlic
- 1" piece lemon rind
- 12 ounce riced cauliflower, frozen
- 3 Tablespoons bacon fat
- 2 teaspoons salt
- 2 Tablespoons MCT oil

Instructions:

1 Preheat oven to 400°F/200°C.
2 Spread riced cauliflower onto baking sheet, drizzle with MCT oil and sprinkle with salt.

3 Bake for about 10 mins.
4 Peel and slice garlic cloves and ginger root. Peel off a slice of lemon rind and cut green onions into 1" pieces.
5 Heat skillet on medium heat. Add bacon fat and aromatics, sautéing until fragrant and tender.
6 Add shrimp and sauté until pink and coiled.
7 Add salt and coconut aminos and stir for 2 to 3 mins. Remove from heat.
8 Serve over cauliflower rice and garnish with sesame seeds, chili flakes, or green onion.

Balsamic-Lemon Chicken

Servings: 6 | Total Time: 35 mins
Nutrition Information
Calories: 592 | Carbs: 3.9 grams | Fats: 37.8 grams

Ingredients:

- ◆ 2 chicken cutlets
- ◆ 5 mushrooms, cremini variety
- ◆ 1/3 cup full-fat coconut milk
- ◆ 1 onion, small
- ◆ 3 Tablespoons butter, unsalted
- ◆ ½ teaspoon each thyme and salt

Instructions:

1. Heat pressure cooker on sauté mode and add 2 Tablespoons butter.
2. While butter is melting, peel and slice onion. Prep cabbage and lemon rind as well.
3. Add cabbage, lemon rind, and onion to pressure cooker, stirring until tender.
4. Add chicken thighs and seasonings (including bay leaves). Cook for about 3 mins, until chicken is brown.
5. Add balsamic vinegar and cancel sauté function.
6. Close lid and switch to pressure cook function, high for 20 mins- or poultry function.
7. Once finished, allow natural release of pressure. Open lid and stir to shred chicken.
8. Serve with zoodles, drizzling with avocado or olive oil.

Chicken with Creamy Mushroom Sauce

Servings: 2 | Total Time: 25 mins
Nutrition Information
Calories: 532 | Carbs: 3.9 grams | Fats: 37.8 grams

Ingredients:

- 2 chicken cutlets
- 5 mushroom593s, cremini variety
- 1 onion, small
- ½ teaspoon each thyme and salt (add more salt if desired)
- 3 Tablespoons unsalted butter
- 1/3 cup coconut milk, full fat

Instructions:

1 Heat cast iron skillet on medium heat. While the skillet is getting hot, slice onions and mushrooms.

2 Once skillet is hot, add 2 Tablespoons butter. Once butter is melted, add the mushrooms and season with salt. Saute until brown.

3 Add onions and cook for about 6 mins.

4 Remove from skillet.

5 Add 1 Tablespoon of butter. Sprinkle chicken with thyme and salt and add to skillet. Cook for 10 minutes, flipping over halfway through.

6 Add mushrooms/onions back to mix and pour in coconut oil.

7 Allow mixture to simmer for 1-2 mins.

BBQ Shredded Beef Sandwich

Servings: 4 | Total Time: 8-12 hours
Nutrition Information
Calories: 872 | Carbs: 6.1 grams | Fats: 40.2 grams

Ingredients:

- 3 pound chuck roast
- 2 teaspoons each salt and garlic powder
- 1 teaspoon each black pepper and onion powder
- 2 Tablespoon tomato paste
- 1 Tablespoon paprika
- ½ cup broth
- ¼ cup apple cider vinegat
- ¼ cup butter
- 2 Tablespoons coconut aminos

Instructions:

1 Cut beef into 2 pieces and trim fat.
2 In small bowl, combine pepper, onion, garlic, paprika, and salt and rub on beef.
3 Place beef in slow cooker.
4 Melt butter in separate bowl and whisk in tomato paste, vinegar, and coconut aminos. Pour over beef.
5 Add broth to slow cooker. Set to low and let cook for about 11 hours.
6 When done, remove beef and switch slow cooker to high to allow sauce to thicken.
7 Shred beef and add back to slow cooker to toss in sauce.

Sesame Salmon with Baby Bok Choy & Mushrooms

Servings: 4 | Total Time: 30 mins

Nutrition Information

Calories: 292 | Carbs: 3 grams | Fats: 16.3 grams

Ingredients:

Salmon

- 4 salmon filets, 4-6 ounces each
- 2 portabello mushroom caps
- 4 baby bok choy
- 1 green onio
- 1 Tablespoon sesame seeds, toasted

Marinade

- 1 teaspoon each ginger and sesame oil
- 1 Tablespoon each coconut aminos andolive oil
- ½ teaspoon each salt and pepper
- Juice from ½ lemon

Instructions:

1. In small bowl, whisk together Ingredients: for marinade.
2. Drizzle half onto salmon and turn to coat. Cover and place in fridge for one hour to marinate.
3. Preheat oven to 400°F/200°C.
4. Prepare veggies by trimming the rough ends off the bok choy and cutting in half. Slice mushrooms into ½" pieces.
5. Drizzle remaining marinade over veggies.
6. Spread on parchment paper- lined baking sheet.
7. Place salmon on lined baking sheet and bake until cooked through, about 18-20 mins

.Quick and Easy Chicken Curry

Servings: 2 | Total Time: 35-40 mins
Nutrition Information
Calories: 575 | Carbs: 5.4 grams | Fats: 30.9 grams

Ingredients:

- 1 pound ground chicken
- 1 Tablespoon curry powder
- 2 Tablespoons coconut oil
- 1 can coconut milk (400mL)
- Salt and pepper, to taste
- ½ head cauliflower, broken up

Instructions:

1 In small pot, melt coconut oil. Add chicken and cook until slightly brown.
2 Add curry powder, salt, and coconut milk and cover. Simmer for 15 mins.
3 Add cauliflower and replace cover. Cook for 5 mins.
4 Season as desired with salt/pepper.

Salmon Curry

Servings: 2 | Total Time: 25-30 mins
Nutrition Information
Calories: 1050 | Carbs: 93.9 grams | Fats: 54 grams

Ingredients:

- 2 Tablespoons coconut oil
- Cream from coconut milk
- 1 pound diced salmon
- ½ onion, chopped fine
- 1 teaspoon garlic powder
- 2 cups diced green beans
- 2 cups broth
- Salt/pepper, as desired
- For garnish: 2 Tablespoons basil (optional)

Instructions:

1 Cook onion until translucent. Add green beans and cook for a few more mins.

2 Add broth and bring to a boil.

3 Add garlic and curry.

4 Add salmon.

5 Add coconut cream and simmer until salmon is cooked (about 3-5 mins).

6 Add salt and pepper as desired.

Pressure Cooker Garlic Butter Chicken

Servings: 4 | Total Time: 45 mins
Nutrition Information
Calories: 403 | Carbs: 2.8 grams | Fats: 23.7 grams

Ingredients:

- 4 boneless/skinless chicken breasts
- 10 cloves garlic, peeled/diced
- 1 teaspoon salt
- ¼ cup ghee
- 1 teaspoon turmeric powder

Instructions:

1. Place chicken breasts in pressure cooker.
2. Add ghee with turmeric, garlic, and salt to chicken.
3. Set pressure cooker to high for 35 mins. Follow the Instructions: that came with the pressure cooker for pressure release.
4. Shred chicken in pot.
5. Serve with more ghee if desired.

Chicken Bacon Burgers with Guacamole

Servings: 8 | Total Time: 25 mins
Nutrition Information
Calories: 249 | Carbs: 4.4 grams | Fats: 14.1 grams

Ingredients:

Burgers

- 4 slices bacon
- 4 chicken breasts
- 2 garlic cloves
- 4 Tablespoons/60 ml avocado oil
- ¼ onion, medium

Guacamole

- 1 avocado, pitted and mashed
- 1 tomato, diced
- ¼ onion, diced
- 2 Tablespoons/30 ml lime juice
- 2 Tablespoons cilantro, chopped

Instructions:

1 Place chicken, onion, and bacon in food process and blend until smooth. You might need to do this in batches. Create patties from the blend.

2 Fry patties in avocado oil, making sure that burgers are fully cooked.

3 Combine avocado, onion, cilantro, tomato, and lime juice to create guacamole.

4 Serve burgers with guacamole.

Keto Beef & Broccoli

Servings: 2 | Total Time: 22 mins
Nutrition Information
Calories: 433 | Carbs: 8.8 grams | Fats: 27.8 grams

Ingredients:

- 2 cups broccoli
- ½ pound precooked beef, sliced thin
- 3 garlic cloves, crushed
- 2 Tablespoons tamari sauce or coconut aminos (or more, as desired)
- Coconut oil

Instructions:

1 Place coconut oil in skillet on medium heat.

2 Add broccoli.

3 Once broccoli has softened, add beef and sauté for 2 mins.

4 Add coconut aminos or tamari sauce, ginger, and garlic.

Egg Roll Bowl

Servings: 2 | Total Time: 26 mins
Nutrition Information
Calories: 432 | Carbs: 12.6 grams | Fats: 13.4 grams

Ingredients:

- 45 ml/3 Tablespoons avocado oil
- 450 g/1 pound pork tenderloin, cut into strips
- 2 garlic cloves, minced
- ½ each onion, carrot, and Chinese cabbage, sliced thin
- 30 ml/2 Tablespoons tamari sauce
- 5 ml/1 teaspoon toasted sesame oil
- Optional: green onion, for garnish

Instructions:

1 Heat avocado oil in frying pan. Add pork and cook until brown.

2 Add carrot, cabbage, garlic, and onions and cook until soft.

3 Add sesame oil and tamari sauce.

4 To serve, garnish with green onions.

Bacon Spinach Mushroom Skillet

Servings: 2 | Total Time: 23 mins

Nutrition Information

Calories: 342 | Carbs: 5.8 grams | Fats: 24.3 grams

Ingredients:

- 6 slices/168 grams bacon, diced
- ½ pound/225 grams spinach
- 1 medium/84 grams mushroom, your choice
- 1 Tablespoon/15 ml tamari sauce
- Salt/pepper, to taste

Instructions:

1 Cook bacon until slightly crisp.

2 Add mushrooms and cook until soft.

3 Add spinach and cook until wilted.

4 Season with salt/pepper, as desired. If you wish, add tamari sauce as well.

Cheesy Chicken & Broccoli

Servings: 6 | Total Time: 55 mins
Nutrition Information
Calories: 370 | Carbs: 3.6 grams | Fats: 22.8 grams

Ingredients:

- 20 ounces chicken breasts, boneless/skinless
- 2 Tablespoons olive oil
- 2 cups broccoli
- 1 teaspoon oregano
- ½ teaspoon paprika
- ½ cup each heavy cream and sour cream
- 1 cup shredded cheese
- 1 ounce pork rinds
- Salt/pepper, as desired

Instructions:

1 Preheat oven to 450°F/232°C.
2 If using fresh broccoli, you'll want to precook it. If using frozen, precooking isn't necessary.
3 Cook chicken breasts in an oiled pan and then shred it.
4 In mixing bowl, combine chicken, broccoli, sour cream, and olive oil. Mix well.
5 Spread chicken/broccoli mixture into an 8x11 baking dish, firmly pressing in an even layer.
6 Drizzle heavy cream and add seasonings such as oregano, salt/ pepper, and paprika. You can choose other seasonings if you prefer.
7 Add 1 cup shredded cheese over the top of the casserole.
8 In zipper bag, add 1 ounce pork rinds and crush. Sprinkle these over the shredded cheese.
9 Bake for 20-26 mins, until casserole is bubbly.

Snacks/Desserts

In this section, you will find 5 low-carb, keto-friendly snack/dessert recipes.

Keto Fat Bombs

Servings: 16 | Total Time: 30 mins
Nutrition Information
Calories: 184 | Carbs: 5.1 grams | Fats: 17.4 grams

Ingredients:

- 8 ounce cream cheese, softened
- ½ cup peanut butter (ket0-friendly)
- ¼ cup + 2 Tablespoons coconut oil
- ¼ teaspoon salt
- ½ cup chocolate chips (keto-friendly)

Instructions:

1 Line baking sheet with parchment paper.

2 Combine salt, ¼ cup coconut oil, cream cheese, ad peanut butter with hand mixer, beating until fully combined. Place in freezer for 10-15 mins to firm up.

3 When mixture is firm, use cookie scoop/spoon to create dough balls about the size of a Tablespoon.

4 Place in fridge for 5 mins to harden.

5 While balls are in fridge, make your chocolate drizzle by combining chocolate chips and other 2 Tablespoons of coconut oil in microwave safe bowl. Microwave 30 secs at a time until melted.

6 Take balls out of fridge and drizzle chocolate over them as desired.

7 Place back in fridge to harden the chocolate, about 5 more mins.

Keto Chocolate Chip Cookies

Servings: 20 cookies | Total Time: 25-30 mins
Nutrition Information
Calories: 188 | Carbs: 5 grams | Fats: 17.3 grams

Ingredients:

- 3 cups almond flour
- 1/3 cup each butter and coconut oil
- 1 teaspoon vanilla extract
- ¾ cup sweetener
- 2 large eggs
- ½ teaspoon each salt and baking soda
- 3 ounces baking chocolate
- ¼ teaspoon cream of tartar

Instructions:

1 Line baking sheets with parchment paper.
2 Preheat oven to 350°F/176°C
3 With a hand mixer, combine butter and coconut oil.
4 Add eggs and vanilla extract. Continue mixing with hand mixer.
5 Add cream of tartar, sweetener, salt, and baking soda, mixing until well-combined.
6 Add almond flour one cup at a time.
7 Microwave chocolate bar in 15 second increments until softened. Then, break apart by placing in plastic bag and crushing.
8 Add chocolate to dough and combine well.
9 Create dough balls and flatten on prepared cookie sheets- leave plenty of room for dough to spread.
10 Bake for 18 to 20 mins until golden brown.

Blueberry Scones

Servings: 8 scones | Total Time: 45 mins
Nutrition Information
Calories: 138 | Carbs: 6.4 grams | Fats: 8.4 grams

Ingredients:

- 2 scoops vanilla protein powder
- ¼ cup each coconut flour and sweetener
- 3 Tablespoons cold butter, cut into small pieces
- 1 teaspoon baking powder
- 1 ½ cups almond flour
- 1 teaspoon baking powder
- ¼ teaspoon salt
- ½ teaspoon baking soda
- 1 teaspoon vanilla extract
- 1/3 cup heavy cream
- 1 egg
- ½ cup blueberries
- Optional: 4 Tablespoons coconut butter (for glaze)

Instructions:

1 Preheat oven to 350°F/176°C.
2 Line baking sheet with parchment paper
3 Add protein powder, baking powder, coconut & almond flours, baking soda, salt, and sweetener to food processer and pulse to combine.
4 Gradually add cold butter, vanilla extract, heavy cream, ad egg, pulsing until dough comes together but is not over-mixed.
5 Fold in blueberries.
6 Scoop onto baking sheet with a ¼ cup measuring cup, creating 8 even mounds. Leaving 2" between each one, form scone shapes with each mound.
7 Bake for 35-40 mins until golden and baked through.
8 If desired, drizzle coconut butter and sprinkle sweetener on tops.

Fudgy Pecan Pie Bombs

Servings: 12 bombs | Total Time 1 hr 5 mins – 2 hrs 5 mins
Nutrition Information
Calories: 13 | Carbs: 1.1 grams | Fats: 1.2 grams

Ingredients:

- ½ cup each cacao butter and coconut butter
- 2 pieces 100% cacao or ¼ cup chocolate chips (sugar free)
- 2 Tablespoons each butter and sweetener
- ½ cup pecans, chopped
- 1 Tablespoon cacao powder

Instructions:

1 Place pecans in small pot and toast over low heat for 3-5 mins, until fragrant and light golden brown.

2 Remove from heat. Cool and then chop roughly.

3 Add remainder of Ingredients: to pot and place on low heat, melting until smooth.

4 Add pecans, and (if needed) adjust sweetener.

5 Remove from heat and pour into silicone molds.

6 Place in freezer for 1-2 hours, until firm.

No Bake Protein Balls

Servings: 16 protein balls | Total Time: 20-30 mins
Nutrition Information
Calories: 96 | Carbs: 7.7 grams | Fats: 4.1 grams

Ingredients:

- ¾ cup keto-friendly nut butter
- 3 scoops keto-friendly whey protein powder
- 3 tablespoons sugar-free chocolate chips

Instructions:

1 In small bowl, mix whey protein powder and nut butter until smooth.
2 Fold in chocolate chips.
3 Place in freezer for 15-20 mins until firm.
4 Using a cookie scoop, form dough into small balls and place on parchment paper lined baking sheet.
5 Place in fridge to set.

PART 3
BONUS: 14 DAY WEIGHT LOSS & MEAL PLANS

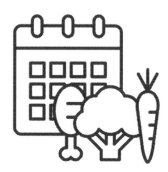

The purpose of this section is to look at a 14-day weight loss and meal plan. If you follow this meal plan very carefully, you will experience the weight loss results that you desire. On the other hand, if you don't follow the plan or change your habits, you're not likely to lose the weight you desire.

Of course, you must know that when you change your eating habits, there are definitely some safety risks that come with this. Therefore, before you make any changes, you must talk it over with your physician. In addition, there are some people who should avoid a keto diet. These are:

1. Women who are pregnant or nursing
2. Those with kidney stones or gallstones
3. Those without a gallbladder
4. Kids who are still growing

Getting started on a new diet can be quite confusing. One of the hardest parts of a new diet/eating plan/lifestyle is knowing what you should cook and what you should avoid. However, if you have a meal plan prepared in advance, it will make your life so much easier. Here, we have provided a 14-day meal plan put together for you. This way, you have 2 weeks to get into the routine and get used to planning your own meal plan.

Each day, we will provide you with a new meal recipe. For the other meals of the day, you can look back at the cookbook we have provided in Part 2 for you. There are some who claim to have lost 30 pounds in two weeks on keto. However, results are more likely going to be somewhere around the 15-20 pounds in two weeks. If you lose more than that, you could end up with health issues.

Day 1

Breakfast:

Salmon Bearnaise Breakfast Bombs

Servings: 2 | Total Time: 15 mins
Nutrition Information
Calories: 701 | Carbs: 0.9 grams | Fats: 68.1 grams

Ingredients:

Bombs

- 4 ounces sliced smoked salmon
- 2 eggs, hard-boiled & peeled
- 2 Tablespoons chopped fresh chives
- 2/3 Tablespoon butter
- Salt/pepper, as desired

Hollandaise

- 1 egg yolk
- 2 Tablespoons salted butter
- 2 teaspoons fresh squeezed lemonade
- ½ Tablespoon water
- ¼ teaspoon Dijon mustard
- Salt, as desired

Instructions:

1. Preheat pan with 2 teaspoons butter.
2. Finely dice salmon and fry half of it until crispy. Set aside.
3. Using a fork, mash eggs well and set aside.
4. Make hollandaise sauce by simmering 2 cups water.
5. While water is coming to a simmer, place 2 Tablespoons butter in microwave and melt. Then, set aside.
6. In heat safe bowl, whisk yolk, mustard, salt, and lemon juice until foamy. Place bowl over the simmering water, but don't let the water touch the bowl.
7. Whisk mixture until it begins to thicken.
8. Add butter slowly and whisk until thickened to desired consistency.
9. Combine raw salmon, mashed egg, chives, and enough hollandaise to create a "dough" consistency.
10. Roll in crispy salmon to coat.

Lunch : Avocado-Chicken-Cucumber Salad

Dinner : Egg Roll Bowl

DAY 2

Breakfast: Breakfast Cups

Lunch:

Taco Bowls

Servings: 4 | Total Time: 30 mins
Nutrition Information
Calories: 360 | Carbs: 18 grams | Fats: 15.6 grams

Ingredients:

Taco Bowl

- 1 pound/450 grams ground beef
- 1 onion, diced
- 6 cherry tomatoes, diced finely
- 1 bell pepper, diced
- 1 teaspoon grated ginger

- 3 garlic cloves, minced
- 2 teaspoons cumin powder
- Dash chili powder
- 2 Tablespoons/30 ml avocado oil
- Salt/pepper, as desired

Rice

- ½ head/300 grams cauliflower, processed into pieces
- 2 Tablespoons/30 ml coconut oil
- Salt and chili powder, as desired

Instructions:

1 Put oil and garlic into large skillet and heat on medium heat.

2 Cook ground beef until almost completely browned.

3 Add onion, tomatoes, and bell pepper. Cook until soft.

4 Add salt, pepper, cumin, ginger, and chili powder as desired, mixing well to incorporate.

5 Make cauliflower rice by sautéing the pieces of cauliflower on high heat for 6 mins in the coconut oil. Season with salt and chili powder as desired.

6 Serve meat over "rice".

Dinner: Salmon Curry

Day 3

Breakfast: BEC Roll-Ups

Lunch: Salmon/Avocado Sushi Roll

Dinner:

Malibu Chicken

Servings: 4 | Total Time: 50 mins
Nutrition Information
Calories: 663 | Carbs: 14.9 grams | Fats: 36.5 grams

Ingredients:

Chicken

- 4 (6-ounce each) chicken breasts
- Salt/pepper, as desired

Dipping Sauce

- ½ cup (240 ml) mayo
- 3 Tablespoons (43 ml) mustard (your preference)
- 1-2 Tablespoons (1/2 to 1 ounce) sweetener

Topping

- ¾ cup (35 grams) pork rinds, crushed
- ¾ cup (60 grams) grated Parmesan cheese
- 2 teaspoons (10 grams) garlic powder
- 1 teaspoon (5 grams) onion powder
- Salt/Pepper, as desired

Top with:

- 8 slices (approx. 6 ounces) deli ham
- 4 slices (approx. 4 ounces) swiss cheese

Instructions:

1 Preheat oven to 350°F/175°C. Place rack in middle position.
2 Crush pork rinds in food processor, or put them in a zipper bag and crush them with a rolling pin or mallet.
3 Spray 9x13 pan with cooking spray.
4 Place chicken on plate and pat dry. Season with salt/pepper.
5 Combine mustard, mayo, and sweetener in bowl.
6 Coat the chicken with ¼ cup of the mayo mixture and set the rest aside for dipping sauce.
7 Combine pork rinds, parmesan cheese, and seasonings. Sprinkle half of this onto the bottom of the baking dish.
8 Add the chicken to the baking dish and sprinkle remaining crumb mixture over the top.
9 Bake until chicken is cooked through, about 35 mins.
10 Remove from oven and add ham and cheese to top.
11 Place back in oven to melt cheese.

Day 4

Breakfast:

Avocado Bun Breakfast Burger

Servings 1 | Total Time: 20 mins
Nutrition Information
Calories: 734 | Carbs: 24.1 grams Fat 65.6 grams

Ingredients:

- 1 medium avocado
- 1 large egg
- 2 thin slices bacon
- 1 slice each red onion & tomato
- 1 leaf lettuce
- 1 Tablespoon (1/2 ounce) mayo
- Salt, as desired
- Sesame seeds, to use for garnish

Instructions:

1 Place bacon in cold pan. Turn stove on and fry bacon.
2 When bacon reaches desired doneness, remove from pan and crack egg in the same pan.
3 Cook egg until it reaches desired doneness.
4 Slice avocado width-wise, remove pit and skin.
5 Fill hole where pit was with mayo.
6 Layer with onion, tomato, lettuce, egg, and bacon.
7 Season with salt and pepper, as desired.
8 Top with other half of avocado.
9 If desired, sprinkle with sesame seeds.

Lunch: Coleslaw Keto Wraps

Dinner: Shrimp Stir Fry

DAY 5

Breakfast: Jalapeno Egg Cups

Lunch

Greek Meatballs over Green Salad

Servings: 4 | Total Time: 30 mins
Nutrition Information
Calories: 382 | Carbs: 3.4 grams | Fats: 24.2 grams

Ingredients:

Meatballs

- 1 lb (450 grams) beef or lamb
- 2 teaspoons (2 grams) oregano
- 2 garlic cloves, peeled/minced
- Handful of mint, chopped fine
- 4 Tablespoons (60 ml) olive oil
- Salt/pepper, as desired

Salad

- Lettuce leaves
- Tomato, cut into wedges
- Lemon, cut into wedges
- ¼ cup chopped flat leaf parsley

Instructions:

1 Preheat oven to 350°F/175°C.

2 Combine ground meat with mint, salt/pepper, garlic, and oregano. Create meatballs.

3 Add oil to large pan and fry meatballs until browned. Transfer to baking sheet lined with parchment paper. Place in oven for approximately 10 mins.

4 Serve over a bed of lettuce and tomatoes. Squeeze lemon juice over the top and garnish with parsley.

Dinner: Chicken with Creamy Mushroom Sauce

Day 6

Breakfast: Avocado Bacon Bombs

Lunch: Tuna Pickle Boats

Dinner:

Keto Meatballs

Servings: 4 | Total Time: 50 mins

Nutrition Information

Calories: 320 | Carbs: 5.4 grams | Fats: 16 grams

Ingredients:

Meatballs

- 1 pound ground beef
- 2 Tablespoons chopped parsley
- 1 garlic clove, miniced
- ¼ cup parmesan, grated (additional for serving)
- ½ cup mozzarella, shredded
- Salt/pepper, as desired
- 1 egg, beaten
- 2 Tablespoons olive oil

Sauce

- 1 can crushed tomatoes (28 ounce)
- 1 onion, chopped
- 1 teaspoon oregano
- 2 garlic cloves, minced
- Salt/pepper, as desired

Instructions:

1. In large bowl, combine beef with parmesan, egg, salt/pepper, garlic, parsley, and mozzarella. Create 16 meatballs.
2. Add oil to large skillet over medium heat. Add meatballs and cook until golden, approximately 10 mins. Remove and drain on paper towel-lined plate.
3. Add onions and cook for about 5 mins.
4. Add garlic and cook for 1 min.
5. Add tomatoes and season with salt/pepper and oregano and mix well.
6. Add meatballs and cover. Simmer until sauce begins to thicken, about 15 mins. Garnish with parmesan cheese, if desired.

Day 7

Breakfast:

Breakfast Pizza

Servings: 10 slices | Total Time: 45 mins
Nutrition Information
Calories: 128 | Carbs: 6.7 grams | Fats: 9.4 grams

Ingredients:

Crust

- 6 egg whites, large
- ½ cup (64 grams) coconut flour
- 1 cup (8 ounces) unsweetened coconut milk
- 1 teaspoon (5 grams) onion powder
- 2 teaspoons (10 grams) each garlic powder and Italian seasoning
- ½ teaspoon (2.5 grams) baking soda

Toppings

- 3 eggs, large
- 1 tomato, sliced thin
- 1 cup (30 grams) spinach
- ½ teaspoon red pepper flakes
- 1 Tablespoon olive oil

Instructions:

1. Prepare baking sheet with parchment paper.
2. Preheat oven to 375°F/190°C.
3. Whisk together coconut milk, seasonings, and egg whites in a large bowl. Fold in coconut flour until well combined.
4. Using a spatula, spread dough evenly onto baking sheet.
5. Bake about 16 mins, or until dough is set.
6. Remove from oven and reduce temp to 350°F/175°C.
7. Brush olive oil over crust.
8. Spread spinach, and then tomatoes.
9. Crack 3 eggs on top.
10. Season with red pepper flakes
11. Bake until egg whites are set, about 12 mins.

Lunch: Zucchini Grilled Cheese

Dinner: Quick and Easy Chicken Curry

Day 8

Breakfast: Cabbage Hashbrowns

Lunch

Thai Chicken Fried Rice

Servings: 4 | Total Time: 30 mins
Nutrition Information
Calories: 467 | Carbs: 9.9 grams | Fats: 35.9 grams

Ingredients:

- 1 head (600 grams) cauliflower, broken up and dried
- 8 tablespoons (120 ml) coconut oil
- 3 eggs, whisked
- 2 (400 grams) chicken breasts, diced
- ½ onion (55 grams), peeled/diced
- 1 bell pepper (120 grams) diced
- 2 garlic cloves (6 grams) peeled/diced
- 2 Tablespoons (30 ml) tamari sauce/coconut aminos
- 2 teaspoons (10 ml) fish sauce
- 1 Tablespoon (5 grams) fresh minced ginger
- Salt, as desired
- Optional: cilantro to garnish

Instructions:

1 Cut up cauliflower into florets to fit into food processor. Pat dry so that your cauliflower rice doesn't become mushy.

2 Process until you have small, rice-like pieces.

3 Add 3 Tablespoons coconut oil into frying pan on medium heat. Add 3 whisked eggs and allow to cook a little bit before stirring. Gently stir, as if you're scrambling- but keep them from getting too clumpy. Once solid, set aside.

4 Cook chicken in separate pan with 3 Tablespoons oil. When completely browned, set aside.

5 Put 2 Tablespoons oil in frying pan and sauté cauliflower rice, onions, and peppers on high heat. Once cauliflower is softened, add chicken and egg. Cook for about 2 mins.

6 Add 2 Tablespoons tamari sauce and fish sauce, ginger, salt (as desired), and garlic.

7 Cook 2-3 more mins and garnish with cilantro when ready to serve.

Dinner: Keto Fried Chicken

Day 9

Breakfast: Blueberry Muffins

Lunch: Keto Taco Salad

Dinner:

Lemon-Garlic Mahi Mahi

Servings: 4 | Total Time: 40 mins

Nutrition Information

Calories: 572 | Carbs: 12 grams | Fats: 19.7 grams

Ingredients:

- ◆ 2 Tablespoons (1 ounce) oil
- ◆ 3 Tablespoons (1 ½ ounces) butter
- ◆ Salt/pepper, as desired
- ◆ 4 (4-ounce) mahi mahi filets
- ◆ ¼ teaspoon (1/4 gram) red pepper flakes
- ◆ 3 garlic cloves, minced
- ◆ 1 pound (16 ounces) asparagus
- ◆ 2 lemons (1 sliced & one zest/ juice only)
- ◆ 1 Tablespoon (1 gram) parsley (additional for garnish, if desired)

Instructions:

1 In large skillet, melt 1 Tablespoon each olive oil and butter over medium heat.

2 Season mahi mahi and add to hot oil/butter, cooking until golden- about 5 mins on each side. Set aside.

3 Add remaining oil to skillet and cook asparagus until tender, about 3-5 mins. Season with salt/pepper and set aside.

4 Add remainder of butter to skillet, and once melted, add red pepper flakes and garlic, cooking for about 1 min- or until fragrant.

5 Stir in lemon zest, lemon juice, lemon slices, and parsley. Remove from heat and add fish and asparagus back to skillet.

6 If desired, garnish with parsley to serve.

Day 10

Breakfast:

Egg Roll-Ups

Servings: 6 pieces | Total Time: 35 mins
Nutrition Information
Calories: 400 | Carbs: 7.3 grams | Fats: 32.9 grams

Ingredients:

- 10 eggs
- ½ cup (250 ml) coconut milk
- Salt and pepper, to taste
- 1 teaspoon (4 ml) mustard
- 8 slices bacon
- 1 cup (48 grams) chives
- 2 handfuls fresh basil leaves
- 1 cup(22 grams) arugula
- 3 Tablespoons (3 oz) mayo

Instructions:

1 Lay bacon on baking sheet, making sure slices do not touch/overlap. Place in oven.

2 Turn oven to 400°F/204°C.

3 Once oven has reached temp, bacon should be par-cooked. Set timer for about 9 mins, which will give the bacon time to crisp.

4 While bacon is cooking, prep remaining Ingredients:.

5 Crack eggs into blender, and add mustard, salt/pepper, and milk. Dice chives and prepare arugula and basil.

6 When bacon is ready, remove from oven and transfer bacon to cutting board and drain fat.

7 Line same pan with parchment paper, making sure that the sides reach the rim- and there is a little extra on the end that you can pull on later. Spray top of paper with cooking spray.

8 Blend egg mixture for 32 seconds.

9 Make sure pan is on a flat surface and pour egg into it.

10 Sprinkle chives and bacon evenly over eggs.

11 Bake for 21 mins, or until edges are golden and eggs are set (there should be no jiggle).

12 Remove from oven and allow to cool for 11 mins.

13 Check to see if eggs are stuck to parchment paper. If not, pick up carefully and place bottom side up on cutting board.

14 If it is sticking, use paper to flip eggs onto cutting board and then carefully peel away.

15 Smear mayo over entire surface.

16 Starting approximately 2" from one end, arrange avocado in vertical stripe. Next, arrange arugula and basil leaves. Then, alternate until you have approximately 1" left on other side.

17 Pick up starting side and pull it over avocado and roll, as if you were rolling a burrito.

18 Once rolled, cut into 2" pieces and serve.

Lunch: Caesar Egg Salad Wraps

Dinner: Balsamic-Lemon Chicken

Day 11

Breakfast: Zucchini Egg Cups

Lunch

Keto Fish Tacos

Servings: 4 | Total Time: 30 mins

Nutrition Information

Calories: 273 | Carbs: 9.5 grams | Fats: 26.7 grams

Ingredients:

Soft Tortilla Shells

- 1 cup (112 grams) coconut flour
- 2/3 cup (5 1/3 ounce) water, lukewarm
- 2 Tablespoons (32 grams) psyllium husk powder
- 4 teaspoons (20 ml) olive oil
- ½ teaspoon (1 gram) baking soda
- 1 Tablespoon (15 ml) olive oil
- Salt, as desired

Fish

- 14 ounces (400 grams) whitefish filets, skinned/deboned
- Salt, as desired
- 2 Tablespoons (14 grams) coconut flour
- 2 Tablespoons (30 ml) olive oil
- For assembly
- 1 lime, juice and zest
- 4 soft taco shells
- ¼ (28 grams) red onion, thin sliced

Cooked fish

- Soft lettuce leaves
- 4 Tablespoons (60 ml) mayo
- Handful chopped cilantro

Instructions:

1 To make taco shells, combine coconut flour, psyllium husk powder, salt, and baking powder in large bowl.

2 In separate bowl, combine egg, water, and 1 Tablespoon olive oil. Add to dry Ingredients: and use wooden spoon to combine.

3 Divide dough into 4 equal portions and roll into a ball. Then, flatten each between 2 sheets of parchment paper. You want them to be approximately the size of a small plate.

4 Heat 1 teaspoon/5 ml olive oil in nonstick frying pan and place one of your dough pieces into the pan. Cook for several minutes, turning it over halfway through. Continue until all 4 shells are cooked.

5 Cut fish into small pieces and coat with coconut flour. Season as desired with salt.

6 Heat 2 Tablespoons (30 ml) olive oil in separate pan and fry fish pieces until golden and cooked through.

7 Make a spread by grating the lime zest into the keto mayo. Spread 1 Tablespoon (15 ml) onto each taco shell and assemble as desired with toppings.

Dinner: Keto Beef & Broccoli

Day 12

Breakfast: Breakfast Sausage Sandwich

Lunch: Dijon Herb Salmon Salad

Dinner:

Taco Casserole

Servings: 6 | Total Time: 1 hour 15 mins
Nutrition Information
Calories: 451 | Carbs: 3.1 grams | Fats: 24.2 grams

Ingredients:

- 1 Tablespoon (15 ml) olive oil
- 2 pounds ground beef
- Salt/pepper, as desired
- ½ onion, diced
- 2 Tablespoons (28 grams) taco seasoning
- 6 eggs, beaten lightly
- 1 jalapeno, seeded/minced (more for garnish, if desired)
- 2 Tablespoons (28 grams) parsley
- 2 cups (8 ounces) Mexican cheese, shredded
- Optional:1 cup (4 ounces) sour cream

Instructions:

1 Preheat oven to 350°F/176°C.

2 Add oil to large skillet over medium heat. Once heated, add onion and cook for about 2 mins, or until softened.

3 Add ground beef and season as desired with salt/pepper. Cook until brown, about 7 mins. Addtaco seasoning andjalapeno, and cook for about 1 min, until spices are lightly toasted.

4 In large bowl, whisk eggs. Add meat and spread into a 2 quart baking dish. Sprinkle with cheese.

5 Bake for about 25 mins, until set.

6 If desired, garnish with parsley, sour cream, and a jalapeno.

Day 13

Breakfast:

Zucchini-Proscuito-Egg Muffins

Servings: 12 muffins | Total Time: 30 mins
Nutrition Information
Calories: 199 | Carbs: 4.5 grams | Fats: 10.1 grams

Ingredients:

- 1 Tablespoon olive oil
- ½ onion, diced
- 2 zucchini, sliced thin
- 3 cloves garlic, minced
- 12 slices prosciutto
- 1 bell pepper, diced
- 1 cup baby spinach, chopped
- ¼ cup parsley, chopped rough
- 8 eggs, large
- ¼ cup coconut milk
- Salt/pepper, as desired

Instructions:

1. Preheat oven to 350°F/175°C.
2. Heat oil in pan on medium heat and sauté onion & garlic for 1 min .
3. Add spinach, parsley, and pepper and continue sautéing until spinach is wilted.
4. In mixing bowl, whisk together eggs, milk, and salt/pepper. When veggies are fully cooked, add them and the zucchini to bowl and stir.
5. Grease muffin tin and line each well with one slice with prosciutto.
6. Ladle egg mixture into muffin tin and bake for 20 mins, or until cooked through.

Lunch: Keto Cobb Salad

Dinner: Pressure Cooker Garlic Butter Chicken

Day 14

Breakfast: Pepper Omelet Cups
Lunch:

Keto Club Sandwich

Servings: 4 | Total Time: 25 mins
Nutrition Information
Calories: 301 | Carbs: 23 grams | Fats: 14.3 grams

Ingredients:

- 1 Tablespoon/15 ml olive oil
- 6 slices keto bread
- 4 leaves lettuce
- 1 (200 grams) chicken breast
- 1 large tomato (180 grams), thinly sliced
- 4 slices (112 grams) bacon, cut in half
- Salt/pepper, as desired

Instructions:

1 Preheat oven to 335°F/180°C.

2 Cook chicken breast in skillet with olive oil until golden.

3 Place on baking sheet. Bake for about 15 mins, or until cooked through.

4 Place on baking sheet and bake until cooked through, about 15 mins.

5 While chicken is in oven, cook bacon in the skillet used to cook chicken until crispy. Remove from skillet and set aside to cool and drain.

6 Remove chicken from oven and allow to cool before slicing into thin strips. Season with salt/pepper as desired.

7 Place 4 slices bread on plates. Add lettuce and tomato. Top with chicken and bacon.

8 Place 2 of the sandwiches on top of the other two. Then, top each with another piece of bread and cut in half to make 4 sandwiches.

Dinner: Cheesy Chicken and Broccoli

EXCLUSIVE BONUS!

Get Keto Audiobook for FREE NOW!*

The Ultimate Keto Diet Guide 2019-2020:
How to Loose weight with Quick and Easy Steps

SCAN ME

or go to

www.free-keto.co.uk

*Listen free for 30 Days on Audible (for new members only)

DISCLAIMER

The opinions and ideas of the author contained in this publication are designed to educate the reader in an informative and helpful manner. While we accept that the instructions will not suit every reader, it is only to be expected that the recipes might not gel with everyone. Use the book responsibly and at your own risk. This work with all its contents, does not guarantee correctness, completion, quality or correctness of the provided information. Always check with your medical practitioner should you be unsure whether to follow a low carb eating plan. Misinformation or misprints cannot be completely eliminated. Human error is real!

Coverdesign: Oliviaprodesign
Coverphoto: Blinovita / depositphotos.com

Printed in Great Britain
by Amazon

65370008R00066